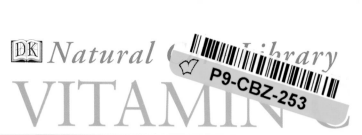

DK *Natural Care Library*

VITAMIN C

BUILDING FLEXIBILITY & FIGHTING INFECTION

P9-CBZ-253

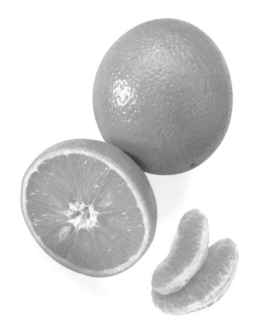

By STEPHANIE PEDERSEN

DORLING KINDERSLEY PUBLISHING, INC.

www.dk.com

CONTENTS

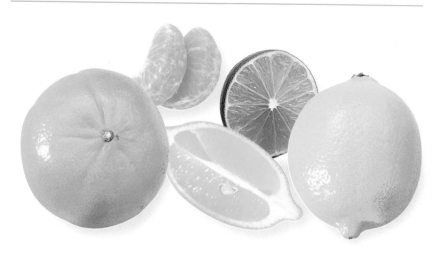

VITAMIN BASICS

The word "vitamin" is a relatively new term. The word first appeared in dictionaries in 1912 and was coined to describe the organic substances in food essential for most chemical processes in the body. Before vitamins were discovered, doctors recommended food itself: carrots (rich in vitamin A) to maintain vision, citrus fruit (high in vitamin C) to prevent scurvy, and whole grains and legumes (abundant in vitamin B_1) to ward off beriberi.

Scientists have identified 13 vitamins that are considered essential for health—essential because the body does not manufacture these nutrients itself. In other words, these vitamins must come either from food or from supplements. Essential vitamins are grouped into two categories: fat-soluble and water-soluble.

Essential fat-soluble vitamins include vitamins A, D, E, and K. These are stored in the body's fat to be used as needed. Because the body stockpiles fat-soluble vitamins, it is possible to take too much of one or more of these vitamins, although this rarely occurs. Vitamin overdose can lead to various symptoms, including headaches and irritability.

The essential water-soluble vitamins are C, B, B_1, B_2, B_3, B_5, B_6, B_{12}, folic acid, and biotin. These are not stored in the body: The body uses just what it needs at any given time and excretes the unused amount in the urine.

Two important points about vitamins. Many people believe that if they take nutritional supplements, they won't have to worry about a balanced diet. But vitamins are just that, supplements. It is important to remember that the human body absorbs vitamins from food more readily than from pills. In addition, science is rapidly discovering dozens of health-supportive phytonutrients in food that work with vitamins to promote health—and these phytonutrients are unavailable in pill form.

Another important point to remember when it comes to vitamins is that you can have too much of a good thing. While large amounts of some vitamins are helpful in specific situations, too much may cause side effects that range from the merely annoying (such as dry skin or sleep disturbances) to the truly dangerous (such as liver damage).

HOW TO TAKE VITAMIN SUPPLEMENTS

• Take vitamin supplements with food to increase absorption. Fat-soluble vitamins should be eaten with food containing some fat.

• If you experience nausea within a half-hour after taking a vitamin, you may not have had enough food in your stomach.

• High doses of vitamins should not be taken at one time. For most efficient absorption, space dosages throughout the day.

WHAT IS VITAMIN C?

Vitamin C is the most widely taken supplement in America. And with good reason. It is responsible for the formation, maintenance, and repair of collagen, the substance that forms the foundation of skin, ligaments, cartilage, vertebral discs, joint linings, capillary walls, and the bones and teeth. Vitamin C stimulates adrenal function and the release of stress hormones, such as norepinephrine and epinephrine. It is the most important water-soluble antioxidant used by humans, meaning it helps prevent oxidation of water-soluble molecules that could otherwise create free radicals—which in turn may generate cellular injury and disease.

Vitamin C stimulates the immune system, helping prevent and treat infections and other diseases. The vitamin is believed to activate neutrophils, the most powerful of the infection-fighting white blood cells. It also seems to increase production of lymphocytes, the white cells important in antibody production and coordination of cellular immune functions. In high amounts, vitamin C has been shown to increase interferon production and thus activate the immune response to viruses, and it is believed to decrease the production of histamine, thereby reducing immediate allergy potential. And that's not all: Current research is studying the link between vitamin C and cancer prevention.

Despite its wide-ranging importance, vitamin C is a recent discovery. The vitamin was first isolated in 1928 by the Hungarian biochemist and Nobel prize winner Albert Szent-Györgyi. That's not to say the effects of vitamin C were unknown: Scurvy, the vitamin C-deficiency disease, has been present for thousands of years. It was first written about around 1500 BC as an illness characterized by lack of energy, gum inflammation, tooth decay, and bleeding problems. Yet it wasn't until the 1700s, when large numbers of sailors were dying of scurvy, that surgeon James Lind discovered that lemons and limes could prevent the deadly disease. British ships began carrying limes for the sailors—hence the origin of the nicknames "limey" and "lime-juicers."

Vitamin C is found in plant foods and is most concentrated in fresh, uncooked foods. It is one of the least stable vitamins, easily oxidized in air, sensitive to heat and light, and quickly destroyed by cooking. The body uses vitamin C in about two hours, and within three or four hours of ingestion, the vitamin leaves the bloodstream completely. This is why researchers suggest taking vitamin C supplements at several intervals rather than once a day.

Interestingly, most animals—with the exception of guinea pigs and primates—produce high levels of vitamin C in their livers. Based both on what these animals produce in their own bodies and the fresh, whole-foods diet of early humans, many authorities feel humans need 600 to 1,200 mg or more of vitamin C daily—quite a bit more vitamin than the current recommended daily allowances (RDA) of 60 mg. Fortunately, maximum levels of the vitamin can be had easily and safely via a diet high in fresh fruits and vegetables.

Natural vitamin C supplements are usually made from rose hips, acerola "cherries", peppers, or citrus fruits. Vitamin C can also be synthesized from high-dextrose corn syrup, much in the way it is made from glucose in animals' bodies. Supplements are available in capsules (both fast-acting and time-released), chewable tablets, effervescents, liquids, powders, and sprays. The vitamin is available as ascorbic acid, L-ascorbic acid, and various mineral ascorbate salts, such as sodium or calcium ascorbate.

FOOD SOURCES

Food is an important, easily digested source of a wide range of
vitamins. The following foods are particularly rich in vitamin C.

Acerola "cherries"
Broccoli
Brussels sprouts
Cabbage
Cantaloupe
Cauliflower
Citrus fruits (all kinds)
Greens (all kinds)
Kiwi
Mango
Papaya
Peppers
Pineapple
Potato
Rose hips
Spinach
Strawberries
Sweet potato
Tomato

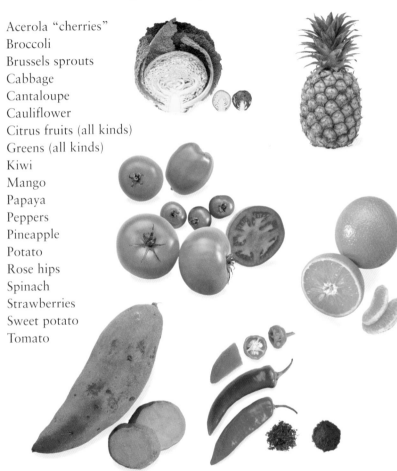

CONSTANT COMPANION

In nature, vitamin C is usually found accompanied by bioflavonoids. These chemical compounds act synergistically with vitamin C to protect and preserve the structure of capillaries, promote circulation, stimulate bile production, lower cholesterol, prevent cataracts, and ward off bacterial invaders. For this reason, we suggest a vitamin C supplement that contains bioflavonoids.

HOW MUCH DO I TAKE?

How many times have you stood in front of the vitamin shelves in your local health food store or pharmacy and compared labels? And how many times have you wondered why one brand offers 60 mg of vitamin C when another boasts 750 mg of vitamin C? Or why another product has 180 mcg of folate when a competing brand features 400 mcg of the same nutrient? And perhaps more importantly, which one is better? When it comes to dosages, there is no magic number. Minimum requirements for nutrients are set by a government board called The Food and Nutrition Board of the National Research Council. These numbers are the recommended daily allowances (RDA) needed to avoid nutritional deficiency diseases such as beriberi, rickets, or scurvy. However, many researchers, medical experts, and health authorities believe that the body needs much higher levels of vitamins for optimum health. And in the presence of illness, pollution, prescription medication, or stress, the body may need still higher levels. For this reason, throughout this book, we suggest a range of vitamin dosages. To determine the best level for you, consult your physician.

Special Needs

While a daily dose of 60 mg of vitamin C is recommended, the following individuals have increased needs for vitamin C:

• Smokers. Cigarette, cigar, and pipe smoking deplete the body of vitamin C.

• Individuals who drink more than two alcoholic drinks a day. Alcohol reduces levels of vitamin C in the body.

• Individuals who eat only cooked fruits or processed fruits and vegetables. Canning, cooking, and freezing break down the vitamin C in foods.

• Individuals who are on analgesics, anticoagulants, antidepressants, oral contraceptives, or steroids. These medications reduce vitamin C levels in the body.

• Individuals who live in polluted environments or who are exposed to secondhand smoke. Pollution and secondhand smoke stress the immune system, depleting vitamin C levels in the body.

• The elderly. With age comes a reduced ability to absorb vitamin C.

• Individuals who are ill or who are scheduled for or have recently had surgery. The body uses increased levels of vitamin C to recover from illness and surgery.

• Depressed or stressed individuals. Both depression and stress have been shown to deplete vitamin C in the body.

VITAMIN C DEFICIENCY

SYMPTOMS OF VITAMIN C DEFICIENCY
- Bleeding gums
- Easy bruising
- Fatigue
- Joint pain
- Poor digestion
- Reduced resistance to cold, flu, and other infectious illnesses
- Slow-healing wounds or fractures
- Weight loss

TOO MUCH OF A GOOD THING
While vitamin C is essentially nontoxic in oral doses, excessive ingestion may cause the following symptoms in some individuals:

- Abdominal bloating
- Diarrhea
- Excessive iron absorption
- Excessive urination
- False positive results to diabetes tests
- Flatulence
- Nausea
- Reduced copper absorption
- Reduced selenium absorption
- Stomach upset

CONDITIONS AND DOSES

ANEMIA

❐ **Symptoms:** Anemia, also called iron-deficiency anemia, occurs when there is not enough iron in the body. Without the proper amount of this mineral, the body cannot produce adequate amounts of hemoglobin. Why does this matter? Hemoglobin is responsible for carrying tissue-nourishing oxygen from the lungs to every part of the body. Without oxygen, the body cannot function properly. A low-iron diet, heavy monthly menstrual flow, pregnancy, lead poisoning, recent blood loss, or poor iron absorption by the body can all lead to anemia. Initial signs are so mild they often go unnoticed: Greater-than-usual fatigue or slight pallor are common symptoms. Later on, the heart rate may grow faster and the sufferer may become winded more easily than usual.

❐ **How Vitamin C Can Help:** One of vitamin C's functions is to help the body absorb and metabolize iron. Iron is a mineral needed to create hemoglobin, the protein in red blood cells. The body doesn't easily assimilate iron, however, and often only minimal to moderate portions of the mineral are absorbed from food and supplements. That said, one study found that consuming 75 mg of vitamin C along with iron-rich food or iron supplements helps the body fully or almost fully incorporate the mineral.

❐ **Dosages:** 75 to 100 mg of vitamin C with bioflavonoids three times daily with meals. In addition, consume five servings of fruits and vegetables daily.

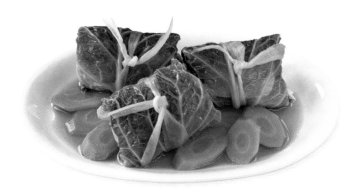

CONDITIONS AND DOSES

ASTHMA

❏ **Symptoms:** Asthma is an inflammation of the airways. It is caused by an allergic reaction and is estimated to affect between 10 million and 14 million Americans. Although not all sufferers are allergic to the same substances, some common triggers are animal dander, dust mites, mold spores, and pollen. When a trigger is inhaled, the body's antibodies react with the allergen, producing allergen-suppressing histamine and other chemicals. Also, chest muscles constrict, the bronchial lining swells, and the body creates more mucus, thus causing difficult breathing, coughing (sometimes accompanied by mucus), painless tightness in the chest, and wheezing.

❏ **How Vitamin C Can Help:** While vitamin C cannot cure asthma, it has been shown to prevent attacks and lessen symptoms during an attack. How does it work? Vitamin C strengthens the immune system, helping it to better fight off allergens. The vitamin is also the primary antioxidant in the bronchi and lungs. This is important because asthma attacks frequently occur when the lungs are under stress from allergens. These allergens produce oxidants that weaken the smooth muscle wall of the bronchi. Vitamin C has been shown by some studies to help squelch the oxidants, preventing them from weakening the lungs and provoking an asthma attack.

❏ **Dosages:** Take 100 to 300 mg of vitamin C with bioflavonoids three times daily with meals. In addition, consume five servings of fruits and vegetables daily.

MISERY HAS COMPANY
If you suffer from asthma, you're not alone. According to the American Lung Association, the prevalence of asthma in the United States since 1982 increased by 49 percent; among children under age 18, the rate rose 78.6 percent. More breath-taking statistics: More than 4,000 people die each year from serious asthma attacks.

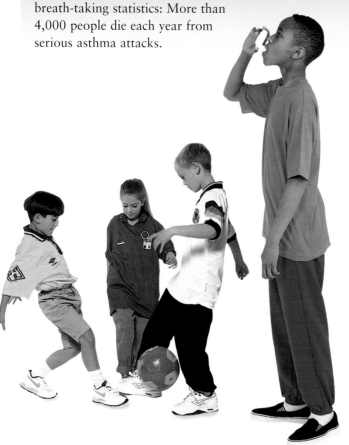

CONDITIONS AND DOSES

RESPIRATORY ALLERGIES

❑ **Symptoms:** A respiratory allergy feels similar to a cold—only with more itchiness. The condition is an immune-system response to a specific airborne allergen, usually animal dander, dust, mold, or pollen. When the allergen is inhaled, an allergic person produces antibodies, which react with the offending substance and prompt the release of histamine. This histamine causes the linings of the nose, sinuses, eyelids, and eyes to become inflamed, which produces a variety of symptoms, including coughing, frequent sneezing, itchiness at the roof of the mouth, itchy eyes, itchy nose, itchy throat, runny nose, stuffy nose, and watery eyes. Interestingly, when a person is allergic to pollen, the allergy is sometimes called hay fever—even though allergies to airborne dander, dust, and mold produce identical symptoms.

❑ **How Vitamin C Can Help:** Vitamin C is an immune-system strengthener that helps the body efficiently fight allergens that have entered it.

❐ **Dosages:** For individuals who are in frequent contact with their "trigger allergen," vitamin C can be used as a preventative. Take 100 to 300 mg of vitamin C with bioflavonoids three times daily with meals. In addition, consume five servings of fruits and vegetables daily.

VITAMIN C TO THE RESCUE!

For those who need further proof of vitamin C's effectiveness against asthma, there is this impressive double-blind study performed in Nigeria during the rainy season—a period when asthma is often exacerbated by respiratory infections. For 14 weeks, 22 test subjects were given megadoses of vitamin C (1 gram per day), while 19 subjects received a placebo. At the end of the study, the vitamin C subjects had less than one-fourth the asthma attacks than the placebo subjects had during the test period, and the attacks they did have were less serious. An interesting note: When the study was over, 13 of the vitamin C test subjects who had experienced no attacks during the study suffered from at least one asthma attack during the eight weeks after the vitamin was stopped.

CONDITIONS AND DOSES

CANCER

❏ **Symptoms:** Cancer occurs when cells begin growing abnormally, forming malignant tumors. These malignant tumors can appear in the breast, the bones, the throat, the brain, the stomach—actually, in almost any area of the body. But why do cells begin acting strangely in the first place? It's believed that exposure to carcinogens causes free radical damage to the cells, which in turn prompts cells to mutate. Common carcinogens include cigarette smoke, fatty foods, industrial chemicals, insecticides, nuclear radiation, pesticides used on food, polluted air, and ultraviolet (UV) light. While cancer symptoms vary widely depending on what part of the body is affected, general signs include blood in the urine or stool, fatigue, hoarseness, indigestion, nagging cough, sores that do not heal, thickening somewhere in the body, and unexplained weight loss.

❏ **How Vitamin C Can Help:** While vitamin C cannot wipe out established cancers, it is a powerful antioxidant. In other words, it has the power to stop free radical damage at a cellular level, thus stopping cancerous cell mutations before they start. As proof of vitamin C's cancer-fighting power, several large-scale epidemiological studies have shown that individuals who eat large amounts of fresh produce rich in vitamin C each day have significantly lower cancer rates than individuals who eat little or no fresh fruits and vegetables daily.

❏ **Dosages:** As a preventative, take 100 to 300 mg of vitamin C with bioflavonoids three times daily with meals. In addition, consume five servings of fruits and vegetables daily.

CANCER TREATMENT COMPANION

When a person gets cancer, the normal course of action is to physically remove as much of the malignant tumors as possible, then follow up with a course of chemotherapy or radiation therapy. Chemotherapy uses drugs or a mixture of drugs to prevent any remaining cancerous cells from spreading. Radiation aims a controlled beam of high-dose radiation at the cancer-stricken area in order to kill cancerous cells. There are downsides to these two types of therapy, including greatly reduced immune-system functioning, which in turn leads to increased susceptibility to colds, flu, and other infectious illnesses. Fortunately, there is help. It's called vitamin C. The vitamin has been found by researchers to increase the immune-system functioning of cancer patients undergoing chemotherapy or radiation therapy, thus strengthening their resistance to a wide range of infectious conditions.

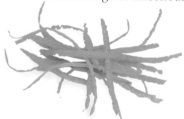
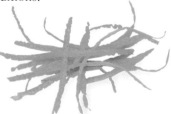

CONDITIONS AND DOSES

CATARACTS

❏ **Symptoms:** Cataracts are one of the leading causes of vision loss in the world; it is believed that 20 million people are blind because of the condition. A cataract is an individual opacity that occurs when large protein molecules aggregate on the normally clear lens of the eye. The lens, a focusing mechanism for the eye, lies just behind the pupil; any clouding of the lens blocks the light needed for sight. Symptoms include blurred vision, impaired vision at night or in dark rooms, difficulty seeing clearly in bright light, and the appearance of halos around lights. Usually a cataract starts in one eye, although both eyes commonly develop cataracts with time. Diabetes, long-term use of corticosteroid drugs, ultraviolet (UV) radiation, and age, are all risk factors for cataracts.

❏ **How Vitamin C Can Help:** Vitamin C is found in high concentrations in the aqueous humor, the watery substance that fills the actual eyeball. It is believed that high concentrations of this powerful antioxidant help protect the eye against the cellular damage that can occur with age, UV exposure, and drug use. This cellular damage often takes the form of cataracts.

❏ **Dosages:** Either as a preventative or a treatment for cataracts, take 100 to 400 mg of vitamin C with bioflavonoids three times daily with meals. In addition, consume five servings of fruits and vegetables daily.

C FOR BETTER SIGHT

At one time, medical experts believed that cataracts leached vitamin C from the body. That view changed, however, with the release of several studies that found just the opposite: Low vitamin C levels were the cause, not the consequence, of cataracts. In one such study recently performed at Tufts University, cataract formation was shown in test subjects to diminish by up to 77 percent with regular vitamin C supplementation.

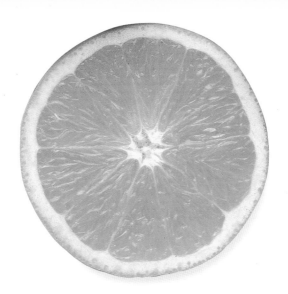

CONDITIONS AND DOSES

ACUTE BRONCHITIS

❏ **Symptoms:** Acute bronchitis is a common illness characterized by inflammation of the bronchi, the breathing tubes that lead to the lungs. Caused by the same virus responsible for the common cold, bronchitis is characterized by constriction of the chest, chest pain, coughing (often with yellowish sputum), difficulty breathing, fatigue, fever, and sore throat.

❏ **How Vitamin C Can Help:** Vitamin C can help fight bronchitis in three ways. First, the vitamin has antiviral qualities, helping to inhibit viral activity in the body. Secondly, the vitamin strengthens the body's immune functioning, helping it fight off infection. Third, vitamin C helps strengthen irritated and inflamed bronchial tissue.

❏ **Dosages:** At the very first sign of illness, immediately take 500 to 1000 mg of vitamin C with bioflavonoids. Follow with 100 to 300 mg of vitamin C with bioflavonoids three times daily with meals. In addition, consume five servings of fruits and vegetables daily. As a preventative, take 100 to 300 mg of vitamin C with bioflavonoids three times daily with meals.

COMMON COLDS

❐ **Symptoms:** The cold is often called the common cold because it is just that: common. In fact, it is estimated that healthy adults get an average of two colds per year. Most colds are caused by a rhinovirus, although in some instances bacteria can be to blame. Symptoms include coughing, nasal congestion, malaise, sneezing, sore throat, and watery eyes.

❐ **How Vitamin C Can Help:** Just how helpful vitamin C is in treating colds is shrouded in controversy. While some research shows that megadoses of the vitamin can quickly squelch a cold, other studies show that vitamin C is only mildly effective. However, the vitamin's strong antiviral and antibacterial ability suggest that it is a safe way to prevent and treat this common illness. Furthermore, vitamin C has been shown in numerous studies to strengthen immune-system functioning, helping the body more quickly and aggressively fight off "cold germs" that have entered it.

❐ **Dosages:** Many researchers believe that vitamin C fights the common cold most effectively when taken as a preventative. Upon exposure to infected individuals, immediately take 500 to 1000 mg of vitamin C with bioflavonoids. Follow with 100 to 300 mg of vitamin C with bioflavonoids three times daily with meals. In addition, consume five servings of fruits and vegetables daily. For treatment of an established cold, take 500 to 1000 mg of vitamin C with bioflavonoids at the first sign of symptoms. Follow with 100 to 300 mg of vitamin C with bioflavonoids three times daily with meals.

CONDITIONS AND DOSES

INFLUENZA

❏ **Symptoms:** Influenza, or flu as it is also known, is caused by a virus that is spread between people via infected droplets of air. Symptoms include coughing, fatigue, fever and chills, headache, muscular aches and pains, nasal congestion, sore throat, and weakness.

❏ **How Vitamin C Can Help:** Vitamin C inhibits viral activity in the body while simultaneously bolstering the body's immune-system functioning. The vitamin has also been shown to lessen muscle aches by strengthening muscle tissue.

❏ **Dosages:** Many researchers believe that vitamin C fights the flu most effectively when taken as a preventative. Upon exposure to infected individuals, immediately take 500 to 1000 mg of vitamin C with bioflavonoids. Follow with 100 to 300 mg of vitamin C with bioflavonoids three times daily with meals. In addition, consume five servings of fruits and vegetables daily. For treatment of an established flu, take 500 to 1000 mg of vitamin C with bioflavonoids at the first sign of symptoms. Follow with 100 to 300 mg of vitamin C with bioflavonoids three times daily with meals.

ANTIBIOTICS: ARE THEY ESSENTIAL?
A recent report published in the *Journal of the American Medical Association* stated that even though antibiotics provide little help for colds, upper respiratory tract infections and bronchitis, doctors still prescribe antibiotics for these conditions. Why? In part, because patients expect their doctors to give them some kind of medication, and many physicians find it easier to oblige than take time out to explain how antibiotics do and don't work. Americans are so enamored of antibiotics that doctors write over 12 million antibiotic prescriptions annually. To learn more about the dangers of antibiotic abuse, contact the Centers For Disease Control and Prevention, 404-332-4555.

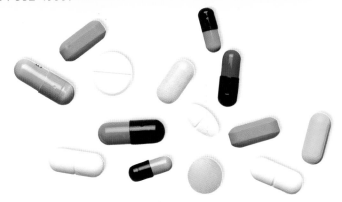

CONDITIONS AND DOSES

CORONARY ARTERY DISEASE

❏ **Symptoms:** Coronary artery disease accounts for about one in two American deaths each year. The disease progresses slowly over the course of years and even decades, but its impact can be instantaneous: In nearly one-third of all cases, death occurs without any previous warning of disease. Indeed, some people have no symptoms, while others may experience chest pain, constriction or a sense of heaviness in the chest, fatigue, pallor, shortness of breath, swelling in the ankles, and/or weakness. Coronary artery disease occurs when cholesterol deposits build up on coronary artery walls. These special blood vessels provide oxygen and nutrients to the muscles of the heart. When they are unable to deliver adequate blood flow, however, the heart muscle begins to weaken, leading to angina (chest pain), congestive heart failure, and heart attack. When it comes to causes, a high-fat diet is most often implicated, although heredity, stress, inactivity, smoking, and alcoholism are also culprits.

❏ **How Vitamin C Can Help:** Researchers have found that vitamin C helps treat and prevent coronary artery disease in several ways: by reinforcing artery walls and the heart muscle with new collagen fibers; by metabolizing cholesterol to bile, which is excreted in the kidneys; and by preventing cholesterol from oxidizing and depositing on arterial walls. Vitamin C also has mild platelet function, keeping blood thin so it can easily pass though clogged arteries.

❏ **Dosages:** As a preventative, take 100 to 300 mg of vitamin C with bioflavonoids three times daily with meals. In addition, eat five servings of fruits and vegetables daily. These dosages can also be taken concurrently with traditional and/or herbal cardiovascular therapies.

One of the better known studies on vitamin C and heart attacks was published in the *British Medical Journal*. The 1984 study looked at the association between concentrations of vitamin C in the blood and risk of heart attack in 1,605 men from eastern Finland who had no evidence of coronary artery disease when the study began. Between 1984 and 1992, seventy of the men had a nonfatal or fatal heart attack. Among men with vitamin C deficiencies, 13.2 percent had a heart attack compared to 3.8 percent among men who were not deficient in Vitamin C.

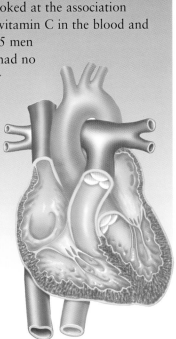

CONDITIONS AND DOSES

HYPERTENSION

❏ **Symptoms:** Hypertension, more commonly known as high blood pressure, is a condition in which blood travels through the arteries at higher-than-normal pressure. This increased blood flow literally wears out the blood vessels, heart, and kidneys and can lead to premature death. What causes hypertension? Cigarettes, alcohol, some medications, and certain illnesses can elevate blood pressure. But by far the most common cause of hypertension is clogged arteries from a high-fat diet. When blood vessels are blocked with fatty deposits, the heart must work harder to move the same amount of blood through them. This in turn increases the pressure at which the blood is pumped. Unfortunately, hypertension is symptomless, leaving many individuals unaware that they even suffer from the condition—until it's too late.

❏ **How Vitamin C Can Help:** Vitamin C cannot cure hypertension. What it can do, however, is help repair and strengthen the arteries and heart by generating new collagen. This makes vitamin C an ideal companion therapy in the treatment of hypertension.

❏ **Dosages:** As a preventative, take 100 to 300 mg of vitamin C with bioflavonoids three times daily with meals. In addition, consume five servings of fruits and vegetables daily. These recommended dosages of vitamin C can also be taken concurrently with traditional and/or herbal cardiovascular therapies.

PENICILLIN BY THE POUND
Since penicillin's debut in 1941, antibiotic production has shot up from 2 million pounds in 1954 to more than 50 million pounds in 1997. Where is all this medication going? Half of the antibiotics produced annually are prescribed for people; the rest are mixed into livestock feed and used as fertilizers for agricultural crops. The downside to this free-flowing penicillin? New, strong, antibiotic-resistant strains of bacteria.

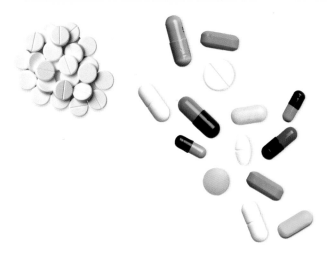

CONDITIONS AND DOSES

CYSTITIS

❏ **Symptoms:** Cystitis is an inflammation of the bladder. Commonly called a bladder infection, the condition is most often caused by *Escherichia coli*, a bacterium that lives in the intestines. Symptoms include cloudy urine that may contain blood, frequent urination, lower abdominal pain, an urgent desire to empty the bladder, and painful burning during urination.

❏ **How Vitamin C Can Help:** Vitamin C and juices rich in vitamin C are often suggested by physicians to help treat bladder infections. Indeed, the vitamin has been shown to combat the *Escherichia coli* bacterium that causes cystitis. In addition, the vitamin is a diuretic that helps promote easier urination by increasing urine output.

❏ **Dosages:** At the first sign of infection, take 500 to 1000 mg of vitamin C with bioflavonoids. Follow with 100 to 300 mg of vitamin C with bioflavonoids three times daily with meals.

LIMIT CHEMICAL EXPOSURE
It's nearly impossible to avoid all chemical toxins in today's world. There's ammonia in cleaning products, chlorine in the water, lead in old paint and pipes, dibromochloropropane in pesticides, carbon monoxide from auto exhaust, and toluene, trichloroethylene, and formaldehyde from printers, photocopiers, and fax machines. Many of these toxins have been linked to allergies, breathing problems, cancer, headaches, infertility, lethargy, lung conditions, reduced attention span, and violence. Ideas for lessening toxins include using environmentally sound dry cleaning, drinking filtered water, purchasing (or making) natural cleansers, limiting the amount of driving you do, and adding a few chemical-filtering plants such as dracaena, chrysanthemum, and weeping fig (Ficus) to your home.

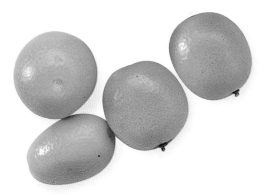

CONDITIONS AND DOSES

OSTEOARTHRITIS

❏ **Symptoms:** Osteoarthritis, also known simply as arthritis, is one of the most common disorders known to humans, affecting up to 80 percent of all individuals over the age of 60. Caused by simple wear and tear of a joint, arthritis is considered a degenerative disease. Symptoms include mild to moderately severe pain in a joint during or after use, discomfort in a joint during a weather change, swelling in an affected joint, and loss of flexibility in the joint.

❏ **How Vitamin C Can Help:** While vitamin C cannot cure osteoarthritis, the vitamin can lessen its severity by helping the body regenerate new joint tissue.

❏ **Dosages:** Take 100 to 300 mg of vitamin C with bioflavonoids three times daily with meals. In addition, consume five servings of fruits and vegetables daily.

RHEUMATOID ARTHRITIS

❐ **Symptoms:** Rheumatoid arthritis is an autoimmune disease in which the body's immune system attacks itself. Though the ailment is not well-understood, it is believed that an unidentified virus stimulates the body to attack its own joints. Symptoms include pain and swelling in the smaller joints of hands and feet, overall aching and/or stiffness after periods of inactivity, and local fever in affected joints.

❐ **How Vitamin C Can Help:** Several recent studies have shown that individuals with rheumatoid arthritis have extremely low concentrations of vitamin C in the blood. These studies suggest that vitamin C may protect against further damage to inflamed joints in two ways: by regulating immune-system functioning, thus lessening the body's attacks on itself; and by helping regenerate new, healthy tissue. Although it isn't known exactly how, vitamin C has also been shown to lessen rheumatoid arthritic pain.

❐ **Dosages:** Take 100 to 300 mg of vitamin C with bioflavonoids three times daily with meals. In addition, consume five servings of fruits and vegetables daily.

CONDITIONS AND DOSES

LOWER BACK PAIN

❑ **Symptoms:** Pain caused by pulled, strained, or weak muscles. Often the pain is so strong that an individual is immobilized.

❑ **How Vitamin C Can Help:** The body uses vitamin C to create collagen, the building block of all the body's tissues, muscle tissue included. Thus, vitamin C works at the cellular level to treat a sore lower back by helping to repair damaged muscle tissue.

❑ **Dosages:** At the very first sign of back pain, immediately take 500 to 1000 mg of vitamin C with bioflavonoids. Follow with 100 to 300 mg of vitamin C with bioflavonoids three times daily with meals. In addition, consume five servings of fruits and vegetables daily. As a preventative, take 100 to 300 mg of vitamin C with bioflavonoids three times daily with meals.

SPRAINED MUSCLES

❐ **Symptoms:** A sprain occurs when a violent twist or stretch causes the joint to move outside its normal range of movement, injuring the muscles and/or ligaments that connect the bones. The result is rapid swelling in the injured area, impaired joint function, pain, and tenderness.

❐ **How Vitamin C Can Help:** One of vitamin C's functions is to help create collagen, the building block of all the body's tissues, muscle tissue included. In the presence of injury, vitamin C works at the cellular level to help repair damaged muscle tissue, thus reducing pain and hastening recovery.

❐ **Dosages:** At the very first sign of muscle pain, immediately take 500 to 1000 mg of vitamin C with bioflavonoids. Follow with 100 to 300 mg of vitamin C with bioflavonoids three times daily with meals. In addition, consume five servings of fruits and vegetables daily. As a preventative, take 100 to 300 mg of vitamin C with bioflavonoids three times daily with meals.

CONDITIONS AND DOSES

BOILS

❐ **Symptoms:** Boils generally occur in individuals with weak immune systems. Known medically as furuncles, boils are inflamed, pus-filled nodules that occur when the *Staphylococcus aureus* bacterium infects a hair follicle and then bores into the skin's deeper layers. The result is localized itching, pain, and redness. A mild fever and swollen lymph glands may also occur.

❐ **How Vitamin C Can Help:** Because boils are contagious, it is important to have a physician lance the boil and remove the infectious pus. Vitamin C has been found in laboratory tests to kill *Staphylococcus aureus* bacteria. In addition, the vitamin strengthens the immune system, enabling it to better ward off bacterial infections. Lastly, vitamin C helps stimulate collagen formation to help repair skin tissue damaged by the boil.

❐ **Dosages:** Take 200 to 400 mg of vitamin C with bioflavonoids three times daily with meals. In addition, consume five servings of fruits and vegetables daily. As a preventative, take 100 to 300 mg of vitamin C with bioflavonoids three times daily with meals.

BRUISES

❒ **Symptoms:** A bruise is a pool of blood that sits directly under the skin. It occurs when blunt force breaks small blood vessels beneath the skin. Though bruises are initially purplish in color, they change to brownish red, then become yellowish and later greenish as blood vessels heal and the body absorbs different constituents of the pooled blood.

❒ **How Vitamin C Can Help:** The capillary-strengthening qualities of vitamin C help speed the healing of broken vessels, thus helping bruises to heal faster. Furthermore, vitamin C is important in preventing bruises. In fact, numerous studies have shown that individuals with low vitamin C intake bruise more easily than individuals who get adequate amounts of the vitamin.

❒ **Dosages:** Take 200 to 400 mg of vitamin C with bioflavonoids three times daily with meals. In addition, consume five servings of fruits and vegetables daily. As a preventative, take 100 to 300 mg of vitamin C with bioflavonoids three times daily with meals.

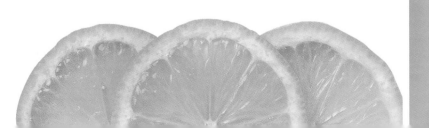

CONDITIONS AND DOSES

BURNS AND SUNBURNS

❏ **Symptoms:** Mild burns caused by hot appliances, heated surfaces, scalding water, or the sun leave the affected area red, inflamed, tender, painful, and sometimes blistered.

❏ **How Vitamin C Can Help:** Vitamin C is a valuable aid in treating burns. How does it work? Collagen-stimulating properties help repair burned tissue, thus speeding healing and reducing the incidence of scarring. In addition, the vitamin is an immune-system booster and antimicrobial, both of which keep burned tissue from becoming infected.

❏ **Dosages:** Take 200 to 400 mg of vitamin C with bioflavonoids three times daily with meals. In addition, consume five servings of fruits and vegetables daily.

THE ANIMAL WAY
Unlike 99.99 percent of all other animals, humans do not manufacture vitamin C in their own bodies. All other animals produce an average of 200 times the human RDA (65 mg) in their liver or kidneys—about 170 mg of vitamin C from glucose per two pounds of body weight. For a human, that would be about 12,000 mg a day.

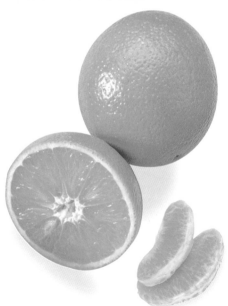

CONDITIONS AND DOSES

STRESS

❏ **Symptoms:** Who doesn't experience periods of stress? Whether caused by increased demands at work, money worries, relationship woes, or something else entirely, stress prompts the body to release what are called stress hormones, such as epinephrine (adrenaline) and cortisol. These hormones help increase blood flow to the muscles and prepare the body for a short period of extreme exertion. However, in times of ongoing anxiety, high levels of these hormones hang around in the body, causing changes in appetite, gastrointestinal upset, headaches, impaired concentration, irritability, muscle tension, sleeplessness, and teeth grinding.

❏ **How Vitamin C Can Help:** Vitamin C stimulates adrenal function and the release of norepinephrine and epinephrine, our stress hormones. However, prolonged stress quickly depletes vitamin C in the adrenals and decreases blood levels of the vitamin. In fact, according to some studies, a body under emotional or physical stress can use vitamin C at up to five times the rate of a nonstressed body. Researchers point to depleted stores of this antioxidant vitamin as the reason why many stressed individuals suffer from a decreased resistance to illness and infection. Thus, extra vitamin C is needed during times of stress to keep the body strong enough to fight off marauding infectious organisms.

❐ **Dosages:** During periodic times of intense stress, take 200 to 400 mg of vitamin C with bioflavonoids three times daily with meals. In addition, consume five servings of fruits and vegetables daily.

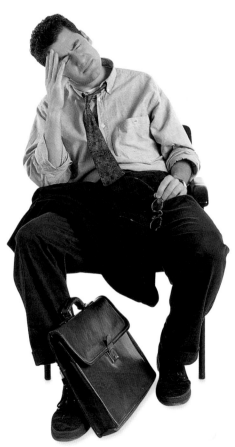

ALTERNATIVE HEALTH STRATEGIES

Herbs, vitamins, minerals—of course these contribute to good health. But creating general well-being involves more than simply taking supplements. Good health has to do with various quality-of-life issues that can aggravate or cause stress, thus harming health. Here are some additional ways to help keep yourself well.

Improve Your Eating Habits

Here are the five main eating strategies people follow; consider finding the most healthful one that works with your lifestyle.

- **OMNIVOROUS**
- **PISCATORIAL**
- **MACROBIOTIC**
- **VEGAN**
- **VEGETARIAN**

Get More Exercise

Whether it's walking or weightlifting, exercise can help you feel better. Try any of these types:

- **STRETCHING**
- **AEROBICS**
- **STRENGTH TRAINING**

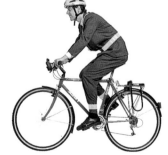

Simple Ways To Ease Stress

In addition to exercise and healthful eating, here are some more techniques—old and new—for easing stress and increasing relaxation.

- GET ENOUGH SLEEP
- MEDITATE REGULARLY
- GIVE UP JUNK FOOD
- ADOPT A PET
- SURROUND YOURSELF WITH SUPPORTIVE PEOPLE
- LIMIT YOUR EXPOSURE TO CHEMICALS
- TAKE YOUR VITAMINS
- ENJOY YOURSELF

ONE-MINUTE STRESS REDUCER

Stress is one of the top health hazards we face today. Unfortunately, it's impossible to go through life without the irritations that make us tense. Fortunately, there *is* something you can do to minimize their power to aggravate you. It's called deep breathing, and it can be done anywhere and anytime you need to calm and center yourself. Here's how to do it:

1. Inhale deeply through your nose.
2. Hold your breath for up to three seconds, then exhale through your mouth.
3. Continue as needed.

Deep breathing pulls a person's attention away from a given stressor and refocuses it on his or her breath. This type of breathing is not only comforting (thanks to its rhythmic quality), but also has been shown to lower rapid pulse and shallow respiration—two temporary symptoms of stress.

GET MOVING

Ask medical experts to name one stay-young strategy and there's a good chance "exercise" will be the answer. And with good reason. Exercise, whether a gentle walk around the block or a full-tilt weight-lifting session, strengthens the heart, lowers the body's resting heart rate, builds muscles, boosts circulation to the body and the brain, revs up the metabolism, and burns calories. All of which can keep a person looking and feeling his or her best. To be effective, exercise must be performed several times a week. Aim for at least three sessions. However, there's more than one kind of exercise. For optimum health, try a combination of aerobic exercise and strength training. And don't forget to stretch before and after each workout!

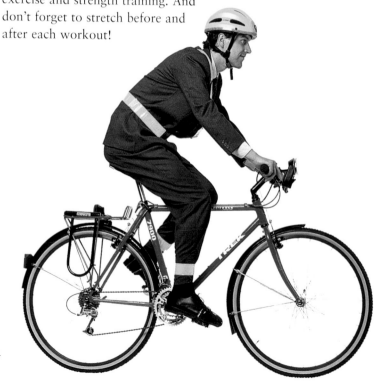

STRETCHING

❏ **What It Is:** Any movement that stretches muscles. Examples include bending at the waist and touching the toes, sitting with legs outstretched in front of you, and rolling your neck. Stretch for eight to twelve minutes before every workout and again after you exercise.

❏ **Why It's Important:** Muscles act like springs. If a muscle is short and tight, it loses the ability to absorb shock. The less shock a muscle can absorb, the more strain there is on the joints. Thus, stretching maintains flexibility, which in turn prevents injuries. Because we often lose our regular range of motion with age, stretching is especially important for older adults to prevent sprains, strains and falls.

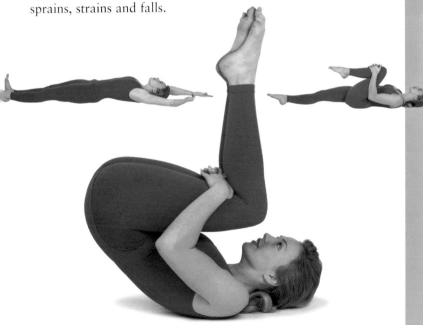

GET MOVING

AEROBICS

❑ **What It Is:** Any activity that uses large muscle groups, is maintained continuously for 15 minutes or more, and is rhythmic in nature. Examples include aerobic dance, jogging, skating, and walking. Ideally, you should aim for three to six aerobic workouts per week.

❑ **Why It's Important:** Aerobic exercise trains the heart, lungs, and cardiovascular system to process and deliver oxygen more quickly and efficiently to every part of the body. As the heart muscle becomes stronger and more efficient, a larger amount of blood can be pumped with each stroke. Fewer strokes are then required to rapidly transport oxygen to all parts of the body.

STRENGTH TRAINING

❐ **What It Is:** Any activity that improves the condition of your muscles by making repeated movements against a force. Examples include lifting large or small weights, sit-ups, stair-stepping, and isometrics.

❐ **Why It's Important:** Strength training makes it easier to move heavy loads, whether they require carrying, pushing, pulling or lifting, as well as to participate in sports that require strength. The exercises are of various kinds. Some require changing the length of the muscle while maintaining the level of tension, others involve using special equipment to vary the tension in the muscles, and some entail contracting a muscle while maintaining its length.

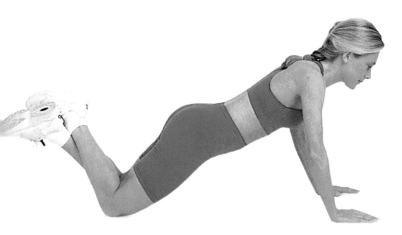

EATING SMART

A balanced diet is the foundation of good health. For proof, just read the numerous medical studies that link healthful eating with disease prevention and disease reversal. These same studies connect high fat intake, high sodium consumption, and diets with too much protein to numerous illnesses, including cancer, cardiovascular diseases, diverticular diseases, hypertension, and heart disease. But what exactly is a balanced diet? Generally speaking, it is a diet comprised of carbohydrates, dietary fiber, fat, protein, water, 13 vitamins, and 20 minerals. More specifically, it is a diet built around a wide variety of fruits, legumes, whole grains, and vegetables. Alcohol, animal protein, high-fat foods, high-sodium foods, highly-sugared foods, sodas, and processed foods are consumed sparingly, if at all.

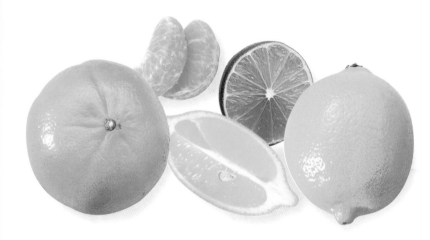

OMNIVOROUS

❏ **On the Menu:** Plant-based foods, dairy products, eggs, fish, seafood, red meats, organ meats, poultry.

❏ **Foods That Are Avoided:** None. Everything is fair game.

❏ **How Healthy Is It?** It depends. Someone who eats eggs, poultry or meat every day, chooses refined snacks over whole foods, and gets only one or two daily servings of fruits and vegetables will not be as healthy as a person who limits meat (the general dietary term for any "flesh foods," including poultry and fish) to two or three times a week, chooses water over soft drinks, and gets the recommended five or more daily servings of fruits and vegetables. Complaints about traditional omnivorous diets revolve around the diet's high level of cholesterol and saturated fat (found in animal-based foods), which increases one's risk of cancer, diabetes, heart disease, and obesity. However, an omnivorous diet can be a healthful one, provided thoughtful choices are made. To keep cholesterol and saturated fat to a minimum and nutrients to a maximum, eat five or more daily servings of fruits and vegetables, choose whole grains over refined grains, enjoy daily legume or soyfood protein sources, and limit the use of animal foods.

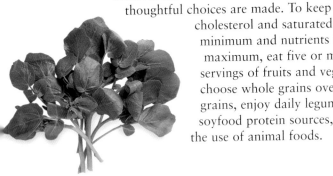

EATING SMART

MACROBIOTIC

❒ **On the Menu:** Plant-based foods, fish, very limited amounts of salt.

❒ **Foods That Are Avoided:** Dairy products, eggs, foods with artificial ingredients, hot spices, mass-produced foods, organ meats, peppers, potatoes, poultry, red meats, shellfish, warm drinks, refined foods.

❒ **How Healthy Is It?** Macrobiotics is based on a system created inn the early 1900s by Japanese philosopher George Ohsawa. The diet consists of 50 percent whole grains, 20 to 30 percent vegetables, and 5 to 10 percent beans, sea vegetables, and soy foods. The remainder of the diet is composed of white-meat fish, fruits, and nuts. The diet's low amounts of saturated fat, absence of processed foods, and emphasis on high-fiber foods, such as whole grains and vegetables, may promote cardiovascular health. Because soy and sea vegetables contain cancer-fighting compounds, macrobiotics is often recommended to help treat cancer. However, critics worry that the diet's limited variety of food can leave followers lacking in certain vitamins and important cancer-fighting phytonutrients.

PISCATORIAL

❐ **On the Menu:** Plant-based foods, dairy products, eggs, fish, seafood.

❐ **Foods That Are Avoided:** Red meats, organ meats, poultry.

❐ **How Healthy Is It?** Like an omnivorous diet, a piscatorial diet is as healthy as a person makes it. Individuals who eat high-fat and highly processed foods, fail to get the recommended daily number of vegetables and fruits, and eschew whole grains for processed grains will not enjoy optimum health. That said, individuals who are conscientious about eating a balanced, varied diet, and who limit fish and seafood intake to two or three times per week, can expect a lower risk of heart disease. Since many oily fish contain omega-3 fatty acids, eating oily fish in moderation has been found to help lower blood cholesterol. Be aware, however, that oily saltwater fish, such as shark, swordfish and tuna, have been found to carry mercury in their tissues; many health authorities recommend eating these varieties no more than once or twice a week. Also, due to overfishing, many fish species are now threatened, including bluefin tuna, Pacific perch, Chilean sea bass, Chinook salmon, and swordfish. For additional information on endangered fish, visit the University of Michigan's Endangered Species Update at www.umich.edu/~esuupdate, or the Fish and Wildlife Information Exchange at http://fwie.fe.vt.edu.

EATING SMART

VEGAN

❏ **On the Menu:** Plant-based foods.

❏ **Foods That Are Avoided:** Dairy, eggs, fish, seafood, red meats, organ meats, poultry. Also avoided are foods made by animals or processed with animal parts, such as gelatin, honey, marshmallows made with animal gelatin, white sugar processed with bone char.

❏ **How Healthy Is It?** A vegan (pronounced VEE-gun) diet can be extremely healthy. Like the vegetarian diet, a vegan diet has been shown by numerous studies to lower blood pressure and prevent heart disease. In addition, the high fiber intake cuts one's risk of diverticular disease and colon cancer. Yet because vegans do not eat dairy products or eggs, they must be more conscientious than vegetarians about either eating plant foods with vitamin B_{12} and vitamin D, or taking supplements of these nutrients.

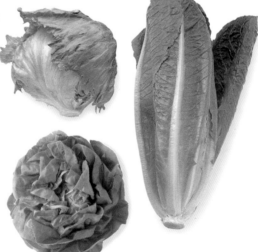

VEGETARIAN

❐ **On the Menu:** Plant-based foods, dairy, eggs.

❐ **Foods That Are Avoided:** Fish, gelatin, seafood, red meats, organ meats, poultry.

❐ **How Healthy Is It?** A vegetarian diet can be very healthy when done right. Fortunately, this isn't hard. Dietary science has debunked theories of "protein combining" popular in the 1960s and 1970s, leaving today's vegetarians to worry only about eating a wide variety of whole foods, including beans, fruits, grains, low-fat dairy products, nuts, soy foods, and vegetables. A varied daily diet insures enough protein, calcium, and other nutrients for vegetarians of all ages, including children, pregnant individuals, and the elderly. A well-chosen vegetarian eating plan has been shown by numerous studies to lower blood pressure, decrease one's risk of breast cancer, and prevent heart disease. In addition, the diet's high fiber levels cut the risk of diverticular disease and colon cancer.

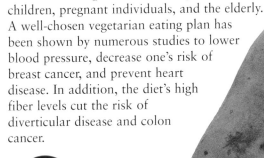

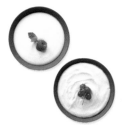

NUTRIENT KNOW-HOW

Vitamins and minerals are known collectively as nutrients. Name a body function, whether carbohydrate metabolism, nerve cell replication, or wound healing, and you'll find one or more of these nutrients at work. The best place to look for vitamins and minerals? In the food you eat every day. Indeed, if you eat a well-balanced diet there's a good chance you'll get all the nutrients your body needs. But if you are ill, pregnant, eat an inadequate diet, drink more than two alcoholic or caffeinated drinks per day,

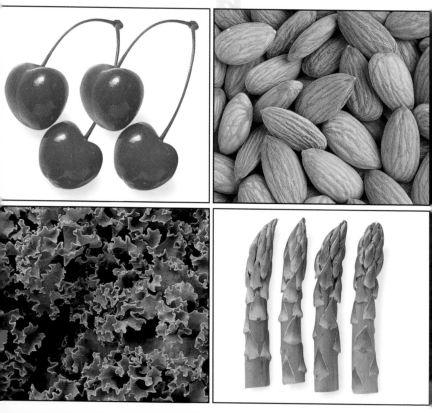

are under stress, are taking certain medications, or have difficulty absorbing certain nutrients, you may need to supplement your diet with one or more vitamins or minerals. Supplements generally come in tablet and capsule form, although some health food stores also carry liquid supplements. Whichever form you choose, doses are measured by weight in milligrams (mg); in micrograms (mcg); or in the universal standard known as international units (IU).

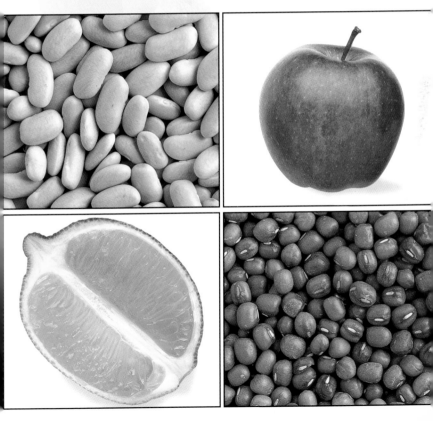

VITAMIN A
(beta carotene, retinol)

What It Does: Vitamin A is found in two forms: performed vitamin A, known as retinol, and provitamin A, called beta carotene. Retinol is found only in foods of animal origin. Beta carotene, a carotenoid, is a pigment found in plants. Beta carotene has a slight nutritional edge, boasting antioxidant properties and the ability to help lower harmful cholesterol levels. Regardless of the form, vitamin A is essential for good vision; promotes healthy skin, hair, and mucous membranes; stimulates wound healing; and is necessary for proper development of bones and teeth.

Recommended Daily Allowance: Men, 5,000 IU (or 3 mg beta carotene); women, 4,000 IU (or 2.4 mg beta carotene).

Food Sources: Orange and yellow fruits and vegetables, dark green leafy vegetables, whole milk, cream, butter, organ meats.

Toxic Dosage: When taken in excess of 10,000 IU daily, prolonged use of vitamin A supplements can cause abdominal pain, amenorrhea, dry skin, enlarged liver or spleen, hair loss, headaches, itching, joint pain, nausea, vision problems, vomiting.

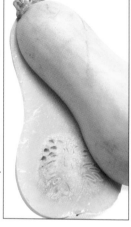

Enemies: Antibiotics, cholesterol-lowering drugs, heavy laxative use.

Deficiency Symptoms: Because vitamin A is fat-soluble, it is stored in the body's fat for a long time, making deficiency uncommon. However, deficiency symptoms include dryness of the conjunctiva and cornea, frequent colds, insomnia, night blindness, reproductive difficulties, respiratory infections.

VITAMIN B₁
(thiamine)

What It Does: Maintains normal nervous system functioning, helps metabolize carbohydrates, proteins, and fats; assists in blood formation and circulation; optimizes cognitive activity and brain function; regulates the body's appetite; protects the body from the degenerative effects of alcohol consumption, environmental pollution, and smoking.

Minimum Recommended Daily Allowance: Men, 1.5 mg; women, 1.1 mg.

Food Sources: Brewer's yeast, broccoli, brown rice, egg yolks, fish, legumes, peanuts, peas, pork, prunes, oatmeal, raisins, rice bran, soybeans, wheat germ, whole grains.

Toxic Dosage: There is no know toxicity level for vitamin B₁.

Enemies: Antibiotics, a diet high in simple carbohydrates, heavy physical exertion, oral contraceptives, sulfa drugs.

Deficiency Symptoms: Appetite loss, confusion, fatigue, heart arrhythmia, nausea, mood swings. Severe deficiency can lead to beriberi, a crippling disease characterized by convulsions, diarrhea, edema, gastrointestinal problems, heart failure, mental confusion, nerve damage, paralysis, severe weight loss.

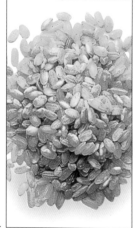

VITAMIN B₂

(riboflavin, vitamin G)
What It Does: Helps metabolize carbohydrates, fats, and
proteins; allows skin, nail, and hair tissues to utilize oxygen;
aids in red blood cell formation and antibody production;
promotes cell respiration; maintains proper nerve function,
eyes, and adrenal glands.
Minimum Recommended Daily Allowance: Men, 1.7 mg;
women, 1.3 mg; pregnant women, 1.6 mg.
Food Sources: Cheese, egg yolks, fish, legumes, milk, poultry,
spinach, whole grains, yogurt.
Toxic Dosage: There is no known toxicity level for this
vitamin, although nervousness and rapid heartbeat have been
reported with daily dosages of 10 mg.
Enemies: Alcohol, oral contraceptives, strenuous exercise.
Deficiency Symptoms: Cracks at the corners of the mouth,
dermatitis, dizziness, hair loss, insomnia, itchy or burning
eyes, light sensitivity, mouth sores, impaired thinking,
inflammation of the tongue, rashes.

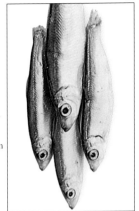

VITAMIN B₅

(pantothenic acid)
What It Does: Helps produce adrenal hormones, antibodies,
and various neurotransmitters; reduces skin inflammation;
speeds healing of wounds; helps convert food to energy.
Minimum Recommended Daily Allowance: 4 mg.
Food Sources: Beef, eggs, beans, brown rice, corn, lentils,
mushrooms, nuts, peas, pork, saltwater fish, sweet potatoes.
Toxic Dosages: There is no known toxicity level for this
vitamin; however, doses above 10 mg can cause diarrhea in
some individuals.
Deficiency Symptoms: Vitamin B₅ deficiency is extremely rare
and is likely to occur only with starvation.

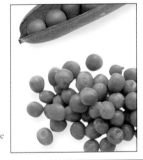

VITAMIN B₆

(pyridoxine)
What It Does: Involved in more bodily functions than nearly
any other nutrient. It helps the body metabolize
carbohydrates, fats and proteins; supports immune function;
helps build red blood cells; assists in transmission of nerve
impulses; maintains the body's sodium and potassium balance;
helps synthesize RNA and DNA.
Minimum Recommended Daily Allowance: Men, 2 mg;
women, 1.6 mg; pregnant women, 2.2 mg.
Food Sources: Avocados, bananas, beans, blackstrap molasses,
brown rice, carrots, corn, fish, nuts, sunflower seeds.
Toxic Dosage: Levels of 2,000 to 5,000 mg can cause
numbness in the hands and feet, and insomnia.
Deficiency Symptoms: Vitamin B₆ deficiency is rare.
Symptoms include depression, fatigue, flaky skin, headaches,
insomnia, irritability, muscle weakness, nausea.

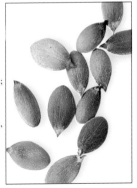

VITAMIN B₁₂

(cobalamin)

What It Does: Regulates formation of red blood cells, helps the body utilize iron; converts carbohydrates, fats, and proteins into energy; aids in cellular formation and cellular longevity; prevents nerve damage; maintains fertility; promotes normal growth.

Minimum Recommended Daily Allowance: Adults, 2 mg; pregnant women, 2.2 mg.

Food Sources: Brewer's yeast, dairy products, eggs, organ meats, seafood, sea vegetables, tempeh.

Toxic Dosage: There is no known toxicity level for vitamin B₁₂.

Enemies: Anticoagulant drugs, anti gout medication, potassium supplements.

Deficiency Symptoms: While deficiency is rare, individuals who do not eat animal products are at risk unless they fortify their diets with plant-sources such as brewer's yeast and sea vegetables. Symptoms include back pain, body odor, constipation, dizziness, fatigue, moodiness, numbness and tingling in the arms and legs, ringing in the ears, muscle weakness, tongue inflammation, weight loss. Severe deficiency can lead to pernicious anemia, characterized by abdominal pain, stiffness in the arms and legs, a tendency to bleed, yellowish cast to the skin, permanent nerve damage, death.

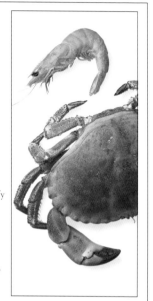

VITAMIN C

(ascorbic acid)

What It Does: Protects against pollution and infection, enhances immunity; aids in growth and repair of both bone and tissue by helping the body produce collagen; maintains adrenal gland function; helps the body absorb iron; aids in production of antistress hormones; reduces cholesterol levels; lowers high blood pressure; prevents artherosclerosis.

Minimum Recommended Daily Allowance: Adults, 60 mg; pregnant women, 70 mg.

Food Sources: Berries, cantaloupe, citrus fruits, broccoli, leafy greens, mangoes, papayas, peppers, persimmons, pineapple, tomatoes.

Toxic Dosage: Doses larger than 10,000 mg can cause diarrhea, stomach irritation, or increased kidney stone formation. **Enemies:** Alcohol, analgesics, antidepressants, anticoagulants, oral contraceptives, smoking, steroids.

Deficiency Symptoms: Bleeding gums, easy bruising, fatigue, reduced resistance to colds and other infections, slow healing of wounds, weight loss. Severe deficiency can lead to scurvy, a sometimes-fatal disease characterized by aching bones, muscle weakness, and swollen and bleeding gums.

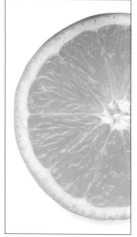

VITAMIN D

(calciferol, ergosterol)

What It Does: Helps the body utilize calcium and phosphorus; promotes normal development of bones and teeth; assists in thyroid function; maintains normal blood clotting; helps regulate heartbeat, nerve function, and muscle contraction.

Minimum Recommended Daily Allowance: Adults, 200 IU (5 mcg); pregnant women, 400 IU (10 mcg).

Food Sources: Dandelion greens, dairy products, eggs, fatty saltwater fish, parsley, sweet potatoes, vegetable oils.

Toxic Dosage: Daily doses higher than 400 IU can lead to raised blood calcium levels and calcium deposits of the heart, liver, and kidney.

Enemies: Antacids, cholesterol-lowering drugs, cortisone drugs.

Deficiency Symptoms: The body naturally manufactures about 200 IU of vitamin D when exposed to ten minutes of ultraviolet light, making deficiency rare. Symptoms include bone weakening, diarrhea, insomnia, muscle twitches, vision disturbances. Severe deficiency can lead to rickets, a disease that results in bone defects such as bowlegs and knock-knees.

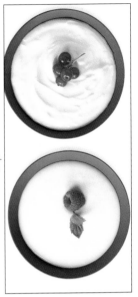

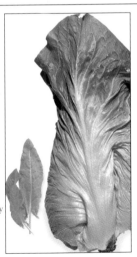

VITAMIN E

(tocopherol)

What It Does: Prevents unstable molecules known as free radicals from damaging cells and tissue; accelerates wound healing; protects lung tissue from inhaled pollutants; aids in functioning of the immune system; endocrine system, and sex glands; improves circulation; promotes normal blood clotting.

Minimum Recommended Daily Allowance: Men, 15 IU (10 mg); women, 12 IU (8 mg); pregnant women, 15 IU (10 mg).

Food Sources: Avocados, dark green leafy vegetables, eggs, legumes, nuts, organ meats, seafood, seeds, soybeans.

Toxic Dosage: Although there is no established toxicity level of vitamin E, the vitamin has blood-thinning properties; individuals who are taking anticoagulant medications or have clotting deficiencies should avoid vitamin E.

Enemies: High temperatures and overcooking reduce vitamin E levels in food.

Deficiency Symptoms: Vitamin E deficiency is rare. Deficiency symptoms include fluid retention, infertility, miscarriage, muscle degeneration.

CALCIUM

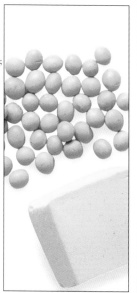

What It Does: Necessary for the growth and maintenance of bones, teeth, and healthy gums; maintains normal blood pressure normal; may reduce risk of heart disease; enables muscles, including the heart, to contract; is essential for normal blood clotting; needed for proper nerve impulse transmission; maintains connective tissue; helps prevent rickets and osteoporosis.

Minimum Recommended Daily Allowance: Adults, 800 mg; pregnant women, 1,200 mg.

Food Sources: Asparagus, cruciferous vegetables, dairy products, dark leafy vegetables, figs, legumes, nuts, oats, prunes, salmon with bones, sardines with bones, seeds, soybeans, tempeh, tofu.

Toxic Dosage: Daily intake of 2,000 mg or more can lead to constipation, calcium deposits in the soft tissue, urinary tract infections, and possible interference with the body's absorption of zinc.

Enemies: Alcohol, caffeine, excessive sugar intake, high-protein diet, high sodium intake, inadequate levels of vitamin D, soft drinks containing phosphorous.

Deficiency Symptoms: Aching joints, brittle nails, eczema, elevated blood cholesterol. heart palpitations, hypertension, insomnia, muscle cramps, nervousness, pallor, tooth decay.

IRON

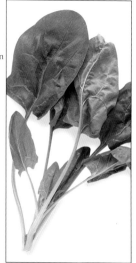

What It Does: Aids in the production of hemoglobin (the protein in red blood cells that transports oxygen from the lungs to the body's tissue) and myoglobin (a protein that provides extra fuel to muscles during exertion); helps maintain healthy immune system; is important for growth.

Minimum Recommended Daily Allowance: Men, 10 mg; women, 15 mg; pregnant women, 30 mg.

Food Sources: Beef, blackstrap molasses, brewer's yeast, dark green vegetables, dried fruit, legumes, nuts, organ meats, sea vegetables, seeds, soybeans, tempeh, whole grains.

Toxic Dosage: Iron should not be taken in excess of 35 mg daily without a doctor's recommendation. In high doses, iron cam cause diarrhea, dizziness, fatigue, headaches, stomachaches, weakened pulse. Excess iron inhibits the absorption of phosphorus and vitamin E, interferes with immune function, and has been associated with cancer, cirrhosis, heart disease.

Enemies: Antacids, caffeine, tetracycline, iron absorption, excessive menstrual bleeding, long-term illness, an ulcer.

Deficiency Symptoms: Anemia, brittle hair, difficulty swallowing, dizziness, fatigue, hair loss, irritability, nervousness, pallor, ridges on the nails, sensitivity to cold, slowed mental reactions.

MAGNESIUM

What It Does: Plays a role in formation of bone; protects arterial linings from stress caused by sudden blood pressure; helps body metabolize carbohydrates and minerals; assists in building proteins; helps maintain healthy bones and teeth; reduces one's risk of developing osteoporosis.

Minimum Recommended Daily Allowance: Men, 350 mg; women, 280 mg; pregnant women, 320 mg.

Food Sources: Apples, apricots, avocados, bananas, blackstrap molasses, brewer's yeast. brown rice, cantaloupe, dairy products, figs, garlic, green leafy vegetables, legumes, nuts.

Toxic Dosage: Daily doses over 3,000 mg can lead to diarrhea, fatigue, muscle weakness, and in extreme cases, severely depressed heart rate and blood pressure, shallow breathing, loss of reflexes and coma.

Enemies: Alcohol, diuretics, high-fat intake, high-protein diet.

Deficiency Symptoms: Though deficiency is rare, symptoms include disorientation, heart palpitations, listlessness, muscle weakness.

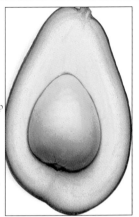

POTASSIUM

What It Does: Maintains a healthy nervous system and regular heart rhythm; helps prevent stroke; aids in proper muscle contractions; controls the body's water balance; assists chemical reactions within cells; aids in the transmission of electrochemical impulses; maintains stable blood pressure; required for protein synthesis, carbohydrate metabolism, and insulin secretion by the pancreas.

Minimum Recommended Daily Allowance: Adults, 2,000 mg.

Food Sources: Apricots, avocados, bananas, blackstrap molasses, brewer's yeast, brown rice, citrus fruits, dairy.

Toxic Dosage: Should not be taken in excess of 18 grams.

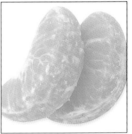

Enemies: Diarrhea, diuretics, caffeine use, heavy perspiration, kidney disorders, tobacco use.

Deficiency Symptoms: Chills, dry skin, constipation, depression, diminished reflexes, edema, headaches, insatiable thirst, fluctuations in heartbeat, nervousness, respiratory distress.

ZINC

What It Does: Contributes to a wide range of bodily processes. Aids in cell respiration; assists in bone development; helps energy metabolism, promotes wound healing; regulates heart rate and blood pressure; helps liver remove toxic substances, such as alcohol, from the body.

Minimum Recommended Daily Allowance: Adults, 15 mg; pregnant women, 30 mg.

Food Sources: Brewer's yeast, cheese, egg yolks, lamb, legumes, mushrooms, nuts, organ meats, sea food, sea vegetables, seeds.

Toxic Dosage: Do not take more than 100 mg of zinc daily. In doses this high, zinc can depress the immune system.

Deficiency Symptoms: Appetite loss, dermatitis, fatigue, impaired wound healing, loss of taste, white streaks on the nails.

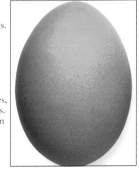

INDEX

ABOUT THE AUTHOR

Stephanie Pedersen is a writer and editor who specializes in the area of health. Her articles have appeared in numerous publications, including *American Woman, Sassy, Teen, Weight Watchers* and *Woman's World.* She has also co-written *What Your Cat is Trying to Tell You: A Head-to-Tail Guide to Your Cat's Symptoms and Their Solutions* and *What Your Dog is Trying to Tell You: A Head-to-Tail Guide to Your Dog's Symptoms and Their Solutions,* both published by St. Martin's Press. She currently resides in New York City.

Picture Credits: Steve Gorton, David Murray, Dave King, Martin Norris, Philip Gatward, Andy Crawford, Philip Dowell, Clive Streeter, Peter Chadwick, Tim Ridley, Andrew Whittack, Martin Cameron

DORLING KINDERSLEY PUBLISHING, INC.
www.dk.com

Published in the United States by
Dorling Kindersley Publishing, Inc.
95 Madison Avenue • New York, New York 10016

Copyright © 2000 by Dorling Kindersley Publishing, Inc.

Editorial Director: LaVonne Carlson
Editors: Nancy Burke, Barbara Minton, Connie Robinson
Designer: Carol Wells
Cover Designer: Gus Yoo

Library of Congress Cataloging-in-Publication Data is available upon request.
ISBN: 0-7894-5196-4